Quick and Healthy Zone Cookbook

Diet for Weight Loss, Health, and Longevity

Deborah B. Gonzalez

Contents

Chapter One

Introduction

The purported health benefits of low-carbohydrate diets have been advocated intermittently over the last century and have enjoyed increasing popularity over the last decade. Although most revolve around the emphatic theme that carbohydrates are to blame for many chronic diseases, their specific ideologies are more variable and, in some cases, quite sophisticated. The Zone Diet phenomenon represents a new generation of modern low carbohydrate food fad with sales placing it among the most popular diet books in recent history. The Zone is a 40 percent carbohydrate, 30 percent protein, and 30 percent fat diet that emphasizes the use of grains and starches in moderation. The precise 0.75 protein-to-carbohydrate ratio required with each meal is promoted to lower the insulin-to-glucagon ratio, which purportedly affects eicosanoid metabolism and, in turn, causes a cascade of biological events leading to a reduction in chronic disease risk, improved immunity, maximum physical and mental performance, increased longevity, and permanent weight loss. There is currently little scientific evidence to back up the claims that diet, endocrinology, and eicosanoid metabolism are linked. In fact, a review of the literature suggests that the Zone Diet hypothesis contains scientific inconsistencies that cast serious doubt on its efficacy.

The Zone Diet, like many fad diets and diet supplements, promises weight loss without hunger. The plan, which was created nearly a decade ago by Dr. Barry Sears, takes a different approach to weight loss by consuming carbohydrates and proteins in precise amounts to promote weight loss. The Zone Diet is a popular fad diet that claims to help slow aging, reverse disease, and increase fat-burning. It was originally designed to control inflammation by switching up your meal plan. It involves changing the macronutrient composition of your diet and prioritizing nutritious, minimally processed ingredients like fruits, vegetables, lean proteins, and healthy fats, just like other weight loss plans. This, according to the diet's creator, can alter your hormone levels and put you in "the Zone," a physiological state that allows you to reap the diet's full benefits.

This diet is focused on helping you control your insulin levels and the rate at which your body uses carbohydrates. As a result, it's very similar to a ketogenic diet, but it's still quite different because you can eat a lot more carbohydrates. Dr. Barry Sears does say that some high-level training athletes may need to consume up to 60% of their daily calories from fats, which is close to keto levels.

The benefits of this diet include its suitability for those with blood sugar problems, diabetes, or a tendency to gain weight quickly on a high-carbohydrate diet. Some people simply cannot tolerate carbohydrates and become sluggish and tired as a result.

consuming them, so this plan would be ideal for them as well. Another benefit of the diet is that, due to its composition, you are unlikely to feel hungry while on it, as all meals will contain a combination of fat and protein (both of which are high satiety macronutrients).

Chapter Two

The Basics and History of the Zone Diet (Chapter 1)

The zone diet is a diet plan developed by Dr. Barry Sears, a researcher at Boston University School of Medicine and the Massachusetts Institute of Technology. It focuses on the ideal state of the body and mind. This is a mental state in which the body feels revitalized and at its most energetic and productive. The term zone was derived from athletes' use of the term "zone peak" to describe the point at which their bodies perform at their best. After his father died of a heart attack in 1970, Dr. Sears, who had studied lipids and their role in the development of chronic diseases in the body, conceptualized the diet. But it wasn't until 1982 that the Nobel Prize jury awarded a research grant to the study of the relationship between hormones known as eicosanoids and the development of diseases such as diabetes, heart disease, and even cancer.

In 1995, the doctor finished his research and published "Enter the Zone," a book that summarized his findings. It became an international bestseller, topping bestseller lists all over the world. It has sold over four million copies to date. Dr. Sears went on to write ten more books on the subject as a result of the book's success. Despite this, critics argue that the theory is flawed because there is no scientific evidence to support it. Although the zone diet is effective in terms of weight loss. Some people are still losing 1.5 pounds per week. There have even been people who have lost weight on the zone diet despite not losing weight on other diets.

Grilled meats, a variety of fruits, and, of course, vegetables are all encouraged in this diet. People participating in the program will eat meals that contain one slice of meat and two-thirds fruits and vegetables. The diet consists primarily of 40 percent carbohydrates, 30 percent protein, and 30 percent monosaturated fats, such as those found in fruits like avocado, guacamole, and macadamia nuts. Carbohydrates can be found in fruits, vegetables, and whole grains. Pasta, rice, and bread are sometimes allowed, but only in small amounts. Protein, on the other hand, is obtained from lean meat and poultry such as chicken and turkey. Fish and soy products can also be consumed.

Chapter Three

Overview of zone diet

When people hear the word diet, the first thing that comes to mind is a brief period of hunger and deprivation in order to fit into a swimsuit, followed by a return to old eating habits. Diet is actually derived from an ancient Greek root that means "way of life." Diet is a lifelong dietary pattern with the goal of achieving some noble goal, such as extending one's lifespan. Diet usually entails self-discipline, but only if the long-term goal is worthwhile. The Zone Diet's goal is to reduce the severity of diet-induced inflammation by reducing the hormonal factors that increase the inflammatory response's intensity. As a result, you'll live longer. Controlling diet-induced inflammation lowers the likelihood of chronic disease development by reducing the amplification of existing unresolved cellular inflammation. As a result, the Zone Diet is an essential first step in improving your Resolution Response. You're either entrusting your future to genetic good luck (which happens occasionally) or abdicating your future to drug companies to manage symptoms of some future chronic disease if you don't have a consistent dietary strategy to reduce diet-induced inflammation. Unfortunately, drugs (even generics) will become increasingly expensive, increasing the likelihood that you will become a walking polypharmacy, taking even more drugs to counteract the side effects of the original drugs. The zone diet is a high-fat, low-carbohydrate diet based on a macronutrient breakdown and a low-glycemic food recommendation. Consume 30 percent dietary protein, 40 percent dietary carbohydrates, and 30 percent dietary fat, according to the macronutrient breakdown. It's usually recommended to eat in "blocks" and to eat about 5 meals per day. Consuming mostly low insulin releasing foods, optimizing satiety, and specific nutrient timing: 5 meals per day with no more than 5 hours between meals are some of the diet's key tenets.

Dr. Barry Sears, a biochemist by training, created the zone diet. The zone diet got its start in the 1970s, when Dr. Sears' father died of a heart attack while he was finishing his postdoctoral fellowship. Dr. Sears was inspired by this life-changing event to investigate the causes of heart disease, and he began to develop a theory about how dietary fat, and how it regulates the body's chemistry and hormones, are important factors in the development of obesity and disease.

Chapter Four

Principles of The Zone Diet

The zone diet is based on the idea that inflammation is caused by insulin and other hormones, and that inflammation is the root of obesity and heart disease. By optimizing hormones, the entire diet is structured to minimize these two things. The zone diet recommends a protein-to-carbohydrate ratio of 0.75 or 3:4 in order to lower the insulin-to-glucagon ratio1. The theory is that eating this ratio optimizes the production and regulation of eicosanoid metabolism, lowering disease risk, boosting weight loss, and extending life.

Calculating the amount of blocks you need to consume per day is required to follow the diet. Throughout the day, each person is given a certain number of blocks. Each person's allowance is determined primarily by biological sex, overall size, and athletic status. For a small female, the total number of blocks per day can range from 10 to 25, while for an athletic - well muscled male, the total number of blocks per day can be as high as 25. The meals are then divided into 5 meals per day, with blocks distributed evenly throughout each meal. Each macronutrient is broken down into blocks: 1 protein block contains 7 grams of protein, 1 carbohydrate block contains 9 grams of carbohydrates, and 1 fat block contains 1.5 grams of fat. An equal number of each block should be included in each meal. A two-block meal, for example, will contain two protein blocks, two carbohydrate blocks, and two fat blocks.

Chapter Five

What Is the Zone Diet?

The Zone Diet is a popular eating plan created by Dr. Barry Sears, an American biochemist and author of the 1995 book "The Zone: A Dietary Road Map." Diet supporters claim that it can help reduce inflammation, which can help with weight loss, slowing the signs of aging, and preventing chronic disease. The diet entails keeping track of your macronutrient intake and sticking to a Ideally, your diet should consist primarily of lean proteins, monounsaturated fats, and low-glycemic-index fruits, vegetables, and whole grains. Keep in mind that the Zone Diet is unrelated to the keto zone diet or the blue zone diet, both of which are weight-loss, longevity, and overall health-improvement eating patterns.

The Zone Diet requires its adherents to consume a specific ratio of 40 percent carbohydrates, 30 percent protein, and 30 percent fat. Carbs with a low glycemic index should be included in the diet because they release sugar slowly into the bloodstream, keeping you fuller for longer. Lean protein and mostly monounsaturated fat are recommended. Dr. Barry Sears, an American biochemist, created the Zone Diet more than 30 years ago. In 1995, he published The Zone, which became a best-seller. Dr. Sears created this diet after losing family members to heart attacks at an early age and realizing that he, too, was at risk unless he could find a way to combat it. The Zone Diet claims to lower inflammation levels in the body. Inflammation, according to Dr. Sears, is the cause of people gaining weight, becoming sick, and aging faster. The diet's proponents claim that reducing inflammation will help you lose fat faster, slow down aging, lower your risk of chronic disease, and improve your performance. The Zone Diet has a specific carbohydrate, protein, and fat ratio of 40 percent carbs, 30 percent protein, and 30 percent fat. Dr. Barry Sears invented it more than 30 years ago.

To provide your body with the fuel it requires, the Zone diet focuses on precisely balancing food intake between protein, carbohydrates, and fats. The Zone program, developed by Barry Sears, MD in the 1990s, teaches you how to use food to achieve a metabolic state in which your body and mind function at their best. The Zone diet is designed to help your body function at its best and reduce your chances of developing dangerous health conditions. A wide range of healthy foods are included in the diet. However, it excludes some foods that most nutritionists consider to be beneficial to a healthy diet, such as grains and legumes. The Zone Diet promises to reduce inflammation and lose weight by structuring meals with 1/3 protein, 2/3 carbs, and a small amount of fat. Experts question some of the 'unfavorable foods' on the list (such as certain fruits), but agree that the diet is generally well-balanced."

Chapter Six

Molecular Basis of the Zone Diet

The Zone Diet is primarily based on hormonal control theory. The body works best on the concept of homeostasis. Think of this concept as a biological thermostat keeping the levels of hormones in the blood within certain operating limits (i.e., a zone). The Zone Diet was developed to keep these hormones in such a zone if you are willing to treat your diet as if it were a drug taken at the right dose and at the right time. In the 1990s the diet debate centered on eliminating so-called "evil" foods. For some like Dean Ornish, it was fat. For others, like Robert Atkins, it was carbs. Neither one understood the impact of the diet on the hormonal balance that affected the generation of pro-inflammatory eicosanoids that caused inflammation, which in turn results in insulin resistance.

In reality, both were partially right and partially wrong. Ornish was partially correct that the wrong types of fat (omega-6 fats and palmitic acid) were very pro-inflammatory. But that was no excuse to throw the baby out with the bathwater by eliminating almost all fat and all animal protein because it also contained fat. Likewise, Atkins was partially correct that consuming too many carbohydrates (especially high glycemic ones like grains and starches) relative to protein would disturb the protein-to-carbohydrate ratio necessary to stabilize blood glucose levels. But by removing most of the dietary carbohydrates, Atkins had also removed the fermentable fiber and polyphenols needed for gut health thereby increasing the likelihood of gut-derived inflammation caused by a leaky gut. At the same time, he was advocating all the benefits of ketosis by eating more fat (especially butter) unaware of the pro-inflammatory properties of saturated fatty acids such as palmitic acid, which is the primary saturated fatty acid in butter. The Atkins diet also perturbs the protein-to-carbohydrate ratio to induce ketosis. One hormonal result consequence of ketosis is to induce the production of excess cortisol that would break down muscle to convert it into glucose for maintaining brain function. The increase in cortisol not only increases insulin resistance but also depresses the immune system.

The Zone Diet was ideally suited to moderate the hormonal extremes advocated by either Ornish or Atkins. You need some carbohydrates, but not too much to maintain a balance of insulin. You also need some protein at every meal, but not too much to maintain glucagon levels that help maintain blood glucose levels. Finally, you also need some non-inflammatory fat at each meal, but not too much, to help release one of the satiety hormones (CKK) from the gut to help maintain satiety as well as provide taste. However, the ultimate controlling factor for insulin levels in the blood is not the levels of carbohydrate in an individual meal, but the degree of insulin resistance a person currently has. That is determined by their levels of cellular inflammation in insulin-sensitive tissues like the muscle, liver, fat cells, and hypothalamus in the

brain. It is insulin resistance that keeps blood insulin levels constantly elevated. This is known as hyperinsulinemia. This same insulin resistance also makes it difficult for the hypothalamus in the brain to correctly receive satiety signals that tell you to stop eating. It is not insulin per se that makes you fat and keeps you fat, but insulin resistance that makes you fat and keeps you fat. Thus, the primary goal of the Zone Diet is to first reduce insulin resistance, and then followed to prevent it from returning. To accomplish both goals you have to maintain a relatively constant protein-to-glycemic load ratio at each meal while restricting calories without hunger or fatigue.

Notice from the diagram that describes the Zone Diet that the shape of protein-to-glycemic load ratio is a bell-shaped curve simply because not everyone is genetically the same. But on the other hand, they aren't that genetically different either.

Chapter Seven

How Do You Follow It?

A typical Zone Diet meal plan should be composed of about 40 percent carbohydrates, 30 percent protein and 30 percent fat. There are two main methods that you can use to estimate your macronutrient intake, including the hand-eye method and the block method. The hand-eye method is the simplest strategy for tracking your Zone Diet macros, which involves dividing your plate into thirds. One-third of your plate should be filled with lean protein foods, such as egg whites, low-fat dairy or skinless poultry, and two-thirds should be composed of carbs with low glycemic indexes, including fruits, veggies or whole grains. A small amount of healthy, monounsaturated fats should also be included, such as olive oil, avocados, nuts or seeds.

Besides paying close attention to what you put on your plate, it's important to monitor when you eat as well. With the hand-eye method, your five fingers are used remind you to eat five times per day and never go more than five hours at a time without eating. In addition to being very simple, the hand-eye method is also flexible and can be a good option when dining out. Another popular method involves tracking Zone Diet blocks, which are calculated based on your specific macronutrient needs. On the diet's official website, it offers a free Zone Diet calculator, which requires you to input your height, weight, body measurements and activity level. It then provides guidelines for the number of protein, carbohydrate and fat blocks that you should aim for each day.

Generally, most women should consume around 11 blocks per day while men should aim for approximately 14 blocks on average. Meals should contain between three to five blocks, and snacks should contain one block, which should be composed of protein, fats and carbs in a 1:1:1 ratio. Here are the amounts of each macronutrient present in a block:

Protein: 7 grams of protein per block Fat: 1.5 grams of fat per block

Carbohydrates: 9 grams of carbohydrates per block

Although this method can be a bit confusing at first, there are many Zone Diet blocks spreadsheet tools and calculators available online to help make it more manageable. The Zone Diet has no specific phases and is designed to be followed for a lifetime. There are two ways to follow the Zone Diet: the hand-eye method, or using Zone food blocks. Most people start with the hand-eye method and progress to using Zone food blocks later, since it is more advanced. You can switch between both methods whenever you feel like, since they each have their own benefits.

The hand-eye method

Chapter Eight

The hand-eye method is the easiest way to start the Zone Diet.

As the name suggests, your hand and eye are the only tools you need to get started, although wearing a watch is also recommended to keep an eye on when to eat. In this method, your hand takes on several uses. You use it to determine your portion sizes. Your five fingers remind you to eat five times a day and never go without food for five hours. Meanwhile, you use your eye to estimate portions on your plate. To design a Zone-friendly plate, you need to first divide your plate into thirds.

One-third lean protein: One-third of your plate should have a source of lean protein, roughly the size and thickness of your palm.

Two-thirds carbs: Two-thirds of your plate should be filled with carbs with a low glycemic index.

A little fat: Add a dash of monounsaturated fat to your plate, such as olive oil, avocado or almonds.

The hand-eye method is designed to be a simple way for a beginner to follow the Zone Diet. It is also flexible and allows you to eat out at restaurants while on the Zone Diet, by using your hand and eyes as tools to choose options that fit Zone recommendations. You can learn more about eating out on this diet here.

Chapter Nine

The Zone food block approach

Zone food blocks allow you to personalize the Zone Diet to your body by calculating how many grams of protein, carbs and fat you can have per day. The number of Zone blocks you should eat per day depends on your weight, height, waist and hip measurements. You can calculate your number here. The average male eats 14 Zone blocks per day, while the average female eats 11 Zone blocks per day. A main meal such as breakfast, lunch or dinner contains three to five Zone blocks, while a snack always contains one Zone block. Each Zone block is made of a protein block, a fat block and a carb block.

Protein block: Contains 7 grams of protein. Carb block: Contains 9 grams of carbs.

Fat block: Contains 1.5 grams of fat.

Here is a detailed guide with different options and how much of each food option is needed to make a protein block, carb block or fat block. You can choose to follow the Zone Diet with either the hand-eye method or the Zone food block method.

Chapter Ten

What Can You Eat?

The Zone diet calls for consuming a precise amount of protein daily based on your percentage of body fat and your activity level. You'll also eat a set amount of carbohydrate-based foods, favoring certain fiber-rich fruits and vegetables over potatoes and grain-based foods such as bread and pasta. Finally, you need to consume fat at every meal. The Zone Diet encourages plenty of lean proteins, low-glycemic carbohydrates and heart-healthy fats. Here are a few of the specific foods that can be enjoyed as part of the diet plan:

Protein

Skinless poultry: chicken, turkey, goose, duck Lean cuts of meat: beef, lamb, veal, pork Seafood: fish and shellfish

Low-fat dairy products: milk, yogurt, cheese Soy products: tofu, tempeh, miso, natto

Egg whites

Carbohydrates

Fruits: strawberries, apples, blackberries, blueberries, melon, oranges, nectarines, plums, peaches, apricots

Vegetables: asparagus, cucumbers, celery, radishes, carrots, tomatoes, cauliflower, broccoli, spinach, kale

Chapter Eleven

Avocados

Whole grains: quinoa, couscous, barley, buckwheat, oats

Nuts: almonds, walnuts, pistachios, pecans, macadamia nuts
Nut butters: peanut butter, almond butter, cashew butter
Seeds: flax seeds, sesame seeds, pumpkin seeds

Vegetable oils: extra-virgin olive oil, sesame oil, peanut oil

Wondering what a typical Zone Diet breakfast, lunch or dinner might look like? Here are some sample meal ideas that you can adjust to fit your needs, along with some simple Zone Diet recipes:

Breakfast:

Chapter Twelve

Lunch:

Egg white omelette with veggies, olive oil and fruit cup
Oatmeal topped with berries and almonds

Greek yogurt with pumpkin seeds and strawberries

Roasted turkey with sautéed kale, sesame oil and fruit cup

Beef and Quinoa Stuffed Bell Peppers with mixed veggies and olive oil Burrito bowl with rice, chicken, avocado, bell peppers and tomatoes

Afternoon Snack: Cottage cheese with sliced plums and walnuts Salad with hard-boiled egg and salad dressing Tuna with crackers and avocado

Chapter Thirteen

Dinner:

Blackened Salmon with Creamy Avocado Dressing with herbed couscous and steamed broccoli

Grilled chicken with side salad, olive oil dressing and sweet potato wedges Marinated tempeh with asparagus, sliced avocado and wild rice

Evening Snack: Hard-boiled egg with whole wheat toast and peanut butter String cheese with mandarin orange and avocado Smoothie with protein powder, berries and almond butter

Foods You Can't Eat

Although no foods are completely off-limits, the Zone Diet recommends restricting foods that are not included on the anti-inflammatory diet pyramid, including many high-sugar fruits, soft drinks and processed foods.

Here are a few other foods that you may want to avoid on the Zone Diet:

High-sugar fruits: bananas, grapes, mangoes, pineapple, dried fruit Starchy vegetables: potatoes, corn, carrots, peas

Refined carbs: white bread, pasta, tortillas, bagels, chips

Processed foods: frozen meals, fast food, cookies, baked goods, pretzels, fried foods Sugary drinks: sweet tea, soda, juice, sports drinks

Caffeinated beverages like coffee and tea should also be limited and swapped for water whenever possible.

General 7-Day Diet Plan

The Zone diet requires you to eat three meals and two snacks consisting of 40 percent carbs, 30 percent protein, and 30 percent fat. Keep in mind, this is not an all-inclusive meal plan and if following the diet, you may find other meals that work best for you. You'll need to calculate your specific protein needs and adjust amounts/portion sizes accordingly.

Day 1: Egg whites scrambled with shredded zucchini and olive oil, slow-cooked oatmeal with blueberries; celery with almond butter, cottage cheese; tuna salad with approved mayo, lettuce, cucumber, grapes; chicken breast with mushrooms, dijon mustard, balsamic vinegar, olive oil, garlic, thyme; smoothie with protein powder, apple, mint, celery, and ginger

Day 2: Low-fat Greek yogurt with mixed berries and almond butter; turkey breast, lettuce, almonds; grilled chicken breast, salad with lettuce, cucumber, olive oil, and red wine vinegar, pear; poached white fish with green beans, lemon, and walnuts, blueberries; cottage cheese with cucumber slices, olive oil, black pepper

Day 3: Egg whites scrambled with pesto, grape tomatoes, and spinach; cottage cheese with diced apple and chopped walnuts; salad with cooked chicken breast, lettuce, chopped apple, walnuts, and balsamic vinegar; baked salmon with slivered almonds; steamed broccoli and cauliflower, strawberries; mixed berries with Greek yogurt and almond butter

Day 4: Scrambled eggs with cheese, Greek yogurt, grapefruit, a half piece of buttered toast, almonds; shredded chicken with salsa, Brussel sprouts, rice; whole wheat pita, avocado, deli chicken, cheddar cheese; sliced steak, roasted carrots, baked potato,

grapes; broccoli; cottage cheese, walnuts, and almonds

Day 5: celery with cream cheese and almonds; low-fat Greek yogurt with raspberries and cashew butter; grilled sirloin steak, salad with mixed greens, cucumber, olive oil, and red wine vinegar, apple; baked trout with olives; steamed asparagus and mushrooms; mixed berries; blueberries, walnuts, and ricotta cheese

Day 6: Eggs, coconut oil, avocado, English muffin, apple; turkey breast, spinach, walnuts; celery with almond butter, cottage cheese; tuna, lettuce, chopped apple, walnuts, and red wine vinegar salad berries; sirloin steak, roasted sweet potato, sauteed mushrooms, broccoli; chicken breast with broccoli, lemon, and walnuts; Strawberry, mint, cucumber, and lemon smoothie with protein powder

Day 7: Scrambled egg whites with pesto, artichokes, and zucchini on whole-grain toast; cottage cheese with chopped kiwi and pumpkin seeds; shredded chicken with buffalo sauce, carrots, celery, rice; whole wheat pita, deli ham, avocado, swiss cheese, tomato; poached cod, potato wedges, peas, lemon butter sauce; Greek yogurt, cashew butter, berries

Men's meal plan using food blocks

For the average man, here is a sample 14-block meal plan. 4 food blocks (breakfast): Scrambled eggs, vegetables, and fruit with turkey bacon.

scrambled eggs (two)

turkey bacon, 3 strips

low-fat cheese, 1 ounce 1 piece of fruit

3 Cooked spinach, 1/2 cup (630 grams) boiled mushrooms (1 cup, 156 grams)

boiled onions (1/4 cup, 53 grams) 1 1/3 teaspoons (6.6 ml) olive oil

Lunch (4 food blocks): Grilled chicken and egg salad with fruit.

3 ounces (84 grams) grilled chicken, skinless 1 hard-boiled egg

Up to 2 heads of iceberg lettuce

1 cup (70 grams) raw mushrooms

1 cup (104 grams) raw cucumber, sliced 1 red bell pepper, sliced

2 tablespoons avocado 1/2 teaspoon walnuts

1 teaspoon (5 ml) vinegar dressing

2 plums

Mid-Afternoon Snack (1 food block): Boiled egg, nuts and fruit.

1 hard-boiled egg

3 almonds 1/2 apple

Dinner (4 food blocks): Grilled salmon, lettuce and sweet potatoes. 6 ounces (170 grams) salmon, grilled

1 cup (200 grams) of sweet potatoes, baked Up to 1 head of iceberg lettuce

1/4 cup (37 grams) tomato, raw\s1 cup (104 grams) (104 grams) raw cucumber, sliced 2 tablespoons avocado

2/3 teaspoon (3.3 ml) olive oil

Pre-Bedtime Snack (1 food block): Cottage cheese, nuts and fruit.

1/4 cup (56 grams) cottage cheese 6 peanuts

1/2 orange

The Zone Diet meal plans break food portions into food blocks, which give you the diet's proportions of macronutrients throughout the day. Sample food block meal plan for women

Here is a sample block meal plan for the average female, with 11 food blocks. Breakfast (3 food blocks): Scrambled eggs with turkey bacon and fruit.

scrambled eggs (two)

turkey bacon, 3 strips 1/2 apple

1 cup (156 grams) (156 grams) mushrooms, boiled 3 1/2 cups (630 grams) (630 grams) spinach, cooked 1 teaspoon (5 ml) (5 ml) olive oil

Lunch (3 food blocks): Grilled chicken and egg salad with fruit.

2 ounces (57 grams) (57 grams) grilled chicken, skinless

1 hard-boiled egg

Up to 2 heads of iceberg lettuce

1 cup (70 grams) (70 grams) raw mushrooms

1 cup (104 grams) raw cucumber, sliced 1 sliced red pepper

2 tablespoons avocado

1 teaspoon (5 ml) vinegar dressing

1 plum

Mid-Afternoon Snack (1 food block): Boiled egg, nuts and fruit.

1 hard-boiled egg

3 almonds 1/2 apple

Dinner (3 food blocks): Grilled salmon, lettuce and sweet potatoes.

4 oz (113 grams) (113 grams) salmon, grilled

2/3 cup (67 grams) of sweet potatoes, baked Up to 1 head of iceberg lettuce

1/4 cup (37 grams) (37 grams) raw tomato

1 cup (104 grams) (104 grams) raw cucumber, sliced 2 tablespoons avocado

1/3 teaspoon (3.3 ml) olive oil

Pre-Bedtime Snack (1 food block): Cottage cheese, nuts and fruit.

1/4 cup (56 grams) cottage cheese 6 peanuts

1/2 orange

A sample meal plan for women is similar to the plan for men, but has 11 food blocks instead of 14.

How to Prepare the Zone Diet & Tips

When following the Zone diet, you're urged to view food as a potent drug that has a powerful impact on your body and your health—more powerful "than any drug your doctor could ever prescribe," according to Dr. Sears. Every meal and snack should have the desired balance of macronutrients—protein, carbohydrates, and fat—that produce an appropriate and favorable hormonal response. First, you'll determine your total daily protein requirement. That amount of protein should be spread evenly throughout the day so that every meal you eat contains a roughly equal amount of protein. Every snack also should contain a smaller amount of protein.

According to Dr. Sears, everyone's daily protein requirement is unique. To calculate yours, first, calculate your percentage of body fat. Then, you use tables provided by Dr. Sears in his book to calculate total mass and lean body mass. Then, you'll balance your protein with carbohydrate foods—again, every meal and every snack should balance protein with carbohydrate, with a ratio of around one-third protein to two-thirds carbohydrate. Finally, you need to eat some fat at every meal. Fat in your diet helps to tell your body that you're full and don't need to eat any more food, and it serves as an important building block of the eicosanoid hormones that the Zone diet is attempting to promote. You need to know how much protein to eat when following the Zone diet since your protein allotment determines your carbohydrate and fat allotment. The key to determining your daily protein requirement is calculating your lean body mass and assessing how active you are. The Zone diet focuses heavily on keeping your body in "the Zone." Therefore, the timing of your daily food intake is critical to accomplish the diet's goals. Specifically, when following the Zone diet, you'll eat three meals a day: breakfast, lunch, and dinner. You'll also allow for two snacks.

Your meals will be evenly spaced throughout the day. Skipping meals is not recommended, nor is loading up at one meal and eating lightly at another. Just as you balance your food intake between protein, carbs, and fats, you'll balance it time-wise. People who are following many other types of diets, such as a gluten-free diet, a vegetarian diet, or a diet that omits certain allergens such as nuts or cow's milk, also can follow the Zone diet with a few modifications:

The Zone diet doesn't require animal-based foods, so if you're a vegetarian or vegan, you can try the Zone diet. However, you should be aware that many plant-based staple foods, including grains and beans, are off-limits on the Zone diet due to their high starch content.

Since the Zone diet omits all grain-based foods (many of which contain gluten), it's easy to make it gluten-free. Therefore, people who have celiac disease or non-celiac gluten sensitivity may find that this diet fits in well with their goals and needs.

If you have diabetes, make sure to talk with your doctor before trying the Zone diet. The program is designed to help balance blood sugar, but people with diabetes could run into trouble by eliminating so many common foods at once.

Sample Shopping List

The Zone diet requires you to purchase a large amount of produce, including leafy greens. This might mean multiple shopping trips to buy fresh produce each week. Unless you have plenty of freezer space, if your lifestyle requires you to consume a lot of protein, you might need to make several trips for lean meats and fresh fish as well. Keep in mind, this is not a definitive shopping list, and if following the diet, you may find other foods that work best for you.

Lean meats (skinless chicken breasts, pork tenderloin) (skinless chicken breasts, pork tenderloin) Low-fat dairy (cottage cheese, yogurt) (cottage cheese, yogurt)

Fresh greens (kale, spinach, swiss chard) (kale, spinach, swiss chard) Fruit (apples, grapes, pears) (apples, grapes, pears)

Healthy fats (olive oil, nuts, natural peanut butter, avocado) (olive oil, nuts, natural peanut butter, avocado) Vegetables (zucchini, celery, cauliflower, broccoli) (zucchini, celery, cauliflower, broccoli)

Lean protein (eggs whites, tofu, protein powder) (eggs whites, tofu, protein powder)

Pros of the Zone Diet

General nutrition: The Zone diet generally follows nutritional guidance that calls for meals primarily carbohydrates, with a smaller amount of protein and a minimal amount of fat. Lean proteins are stressed, and the diet encourages you to consume lots of vegetables and fruit. Sugary drinks and other "junk food," such as candy and chips, are eliminated.

Flexibility: Since the diet allows such a wide variety of foods, it's pretty flexible. People who have other dietary restrictions should find it relatively simple to adapt. You will need to eat similarly sized meals three times per day, but many people already do this, so it won't be a significant change. Meal planning also isn't too tricky since many food combinations will work.

Healthy protein sources: The protein sources consumed on the Zone diet come from lean meats, tofu, egg whites, and low-fat dairy. Higher fat meats are consumed much less, leaving room in the diet for healthier unsaturated fats. Eating a higher-protein diet can prevent muscle loss, increase calorie burn, and keep you feeling full. And limiting saturated fats can improve cholesterol levels and overall heart health.

Cons of the Zone Diet

Difficult to sustain: Some people may find sticking to the Zone diet difficult because of the specific meal components. It is not easy to be sure you are eating the correct amount of protein, carbohydrates, and fats at each meal, especially if you are not at home. Some people may feel deprived due to the limited food choices, making a long-term commitment to this diet less likely.

Complicated tracking: Most diets call for tracking something—calories, carbs, or fat grams. The Zone diet is especially tricky since you'll need to count protein, fat, and carb grams all at once and make sure you consume the right quantities of each.

Unsubstantiated claims: Although the Zone diet is touted as one that can help you ward off serious chronic health conditions such as heart disease, diabetes, and cancer, people who already have been diagnosed with those conditions should talk to their doctors about whether the food restrictions in the diet are suitable for them.

Lacking fiber: The Zone diet eliminates many healthy food choices, such as whole- grain bread, cereal, pasta, beans and legumes, and some fruits. You may find it's challenging to get enough dietary fiber on this diet simply because it places so many good fiber choices off-limits. Fiber has been shown to help prevent and manage type 2 diabetes, cardiovascular disease, and some cancers. 3

Is the Zone Diet a Healthy Choice for You?

Although the Zone diet gets relatively good marks from nutritionists, it doesn't match up well with dietary recommendations from the U.S. Department of Agriculture (USDA) (USDA). The USDA's advice, outlined in the agency's MyPlate tool, calls for you to fill half of your plate with fruits and vegetables and the other half with protein and grains or starchy vegetables. Specific daily amounts are based on gender, physical activity, height, weight, and goals (such as a desire to gain, maintain, or lose weight) (such as a desire to gain, maintain, or lose weight). The protein amounts are similar between the USDA and the Zone diet, but the Zone diet eliminates grain products. In terms of calorie intake, the Zone diet matches the USDA recommendations reasonably closely. Since the Zone diet is designed more to improve your health (with possible weight loss a bonus, not the goal), it doesn't focus on cutting calories substantially. According to Barry Sears, MD, "In the Zone, you'll enjoy optimal body function: freedom from hunger, greater energy, and physical performance, as well as improved mental focus and productivity." Since the diet consists of many healthy whole foods, this may well be true for you, but keep in mind that these claims have not been substantiated and this diet may not meet your specific needs. Speak to your doctor to see if the Zone diet is right for you.

How It Works

According to the diet, since carbohydrates and proteins are the determining nutrients for hormone activity, eating them in perfect combination is the most important rule. As with other low carbohydrate diets, the diet follows an average 40-30-30 ratio of macronutrient intake: 40 percent of caloric intake is complex carbohydrates, 30 percent of intake is protein and 30 percent of intake is fat. In order to achieve the "euphoria," there are favorable and unfavorable food lists from which to choose carbohydrate-, protein- and fat-containing foods. The program attempts to simplify the selection process and the counting of grams by using a "block" system. In general, the system identifies and recommends healthful sources of protein, fat and carbohydrate. For example, chicken breast and turkey breast are preferred over fattier meats such as bacon and pepperoni. Preferred carbohydrates include all vegetables and fruits that are not starchy, hence corn and potatoes are unfavorable choices.

According to the creator of the diet, following this simple eating pattern can alter your hormone levels and allow you to enter "the Zone," a physiological state that helps reduce levels of inflammation throughout the body. In addition to ramping up weight loss, maintaining this physiological state can also optimize cognitive health, slow signs of aging and boost the body's natural fat-burning abilities. In order to determine whether or not you're in "the Zone," Dr. Barry recommends testing your levels of three clinical markers, including:

Triglyceride (TG)/high-density lipoprotein (HDL) cholesterol ratio Arachidonic acid (AA)/eicosapentaenoic acid (EPA) ratio Hemoglobin A1C

If these three levels are within range, the body is said to be in "the Zone," meaning that you are able to reap the full rewards of the diet. The Zone Diet claims to optimize your hormones to allow your body to enter a state called "the Zone." This is where your body is optimized to control inflammation from your diet.

The alleged advantages of being in "the Zone" are: Losing extra body fat as fast as possible Maintaining wellness into older age Slowing down the rate of aging Performing better and thinking faster

Dr. Sears recommends testing three blood values to determine whether you are in "the Zone."

TG/HDL ratio

This is the ratio of "bad" fats known as triglycerides to "good" HDL cholesterol in your blood. A lower value means you have more good cholesterol, which is healthier. The Zone Diet recommends less than 1 as a good value, which is low. A high number for your TG/HDL ratio increases your risk of heart disease. Your ratio for TG/HDL must be tested by a health care professional, such as your doctor.

AA/EPA ratio

This is the ratio of omega-6 to omega-3 fats in your body. A lower value means you have more omega-3 fat in your blood, which is anti-inflammatory. The Zone Diet recommends a value between 1.5–3, which is low. A high number for your AA/EPA ratio is linked with a higher risk of depression, obesity and other chronic diseases. You can test your ratio for AA/EPA at home with a kit purchased on the Zone Diet website.

HbA1c, also known as glycated hemoglobin

This is a marker of your average blood sugar levels over the preceding three months. A lower value means you have less sugar in your blood. The Zone Diet recommends a value of less than 5 percent , which is low. A higher HbA1c is linked to a higher risk of diabetes. Your HbA1c must be tested by a health care professional, such as your doctor.

Supplements recommended

The Zone Diet recommends that you take omega-3 supplements, such as fish oil, to maximize health benefits. They decrease the "bad" LDL cholesterol in your body, and may reduce your risk of other chronic health diseases. The Zone Diet also recommends taking polyphenol supplements, which are molecules found in plants that have antioxidant properties. The evidence behind polyphenols isgrapes; broccoli; cottage cheese, walnuts, and almonds

Day 5: celery with cream cheese and almonds; low-fat Greek yogurt with raspberries and cashew butter; grilled sirloin steak, salad with mixed greens, cucumber, olive oil, and red wine vinegar, apple; baked trout with olives; steamed asparagus and mushrooms; mixed berries; blueberries, walnuts, and ricotta cheese

Day 6: Eggs, coconut oil, avocado, English muffin, apple; turkey breast, spinach, walnuts; celery with almond butter, cottage cheese; tuna, lettuce, chopped apple, walnuts, and red wine vinegar salad berries; sirloin steak, roasted sweet potato, sauteed mushrooms, broccoli; chicken breast with broccoli, lemon, and walnuts; Strawberry, mint, cucumber, and lemon smoothie with protein powder

Day 7: Scrambled egg whites with pesto, artichokes, and zucchini on whole-grain toast; cottage cheese with chopped kiwi and pumpkin seeds; shredded chicken with buffalo sauce, carrots, celery, rice; whole wheat pita, deli ham, avocado, swiss cheese, tomato; poached cod, potato wedges, peas, lemon butter sauce; Greek yogurt, cashew butter, berries

Men's meal plan using food blocks

For the average man, here is a sample 14-block meal plan. 4 food blocks (breakfast): Scrambled eggs, vegetables, and fruit with turkey bacon.

scrambled eggs (two)

turkey bacon, 3 strips

low-fat cheese, 1 ounce 1 piece of fruit

3 Cooked spinach, 1/2 cup (630 grams) boiled mushrooms (1 cup, 156 grams)

boiled onions (1/4 cup, 53 grams) 1 1/3 teaspoons (6.6 ml) olive oil

Lunch (4 food blocks): Grilled chicken and egg salad with fruit.

3 ounces (84 grams) grilled chicken, skinless 1 hard-boiled egg

Up to 2 heads of iceberg lettuce

1 cup (70 grams) raw mushrooms

1 cup (104 grams) raw cucumber, sliced 1 red bell pepper, sliced

2 tablespoons avocado 1/2 teaspoon walnuts

1 teaspoon (5 ml) vinegar dressing

2 plums

Mid-Afternoon Snack (1 food block): Boiled egg, nuts and fruit.

1 hard-boiled egg

3 almonds 1/2 apple

Dinner (4 food blocks): Grilled salmon, lettuce and sweet potatoes. 6 ounces (170 grams) salmon, grilled

1 cup (200 grams) of sweet potatoes, baked Up to 1 head of iceberg lettuce

1/4 cup (37 grams) tomato, raw\s1 cup (104 grams) (104 grams) raw cucumber, sliced 2 tablespoons avocado

2/3 teaspoon (3.3 ml) olive oil

Pre-Bedtime Snack (1 food block): Cottage cheese, nuts and fruit.

1/4 cup (56 grams) cottage cheese 6 peanuts

1/2 orange

The Zone Diet meal plans break food portions into food blocks, which give you the diet's proportions of macronutrients throughout the day. Sample food block meal plan for women

Here is a sample block meal plan for the average female, with 11 food blocks. Breakfast (3 food blocks): Scrambled eggs with turkey bacon and fruit.

scrambled eggs (two)

turkey bacon, 3 strips 1/2 apple

1 cup (156 grams) (156 grams) mushrooms, boiled 3 1/2 cups (630 grams) (630 grams) spinach, cooked 1 teaspoon (5 ml) (5 ml) olive oil

Lunch (3 food blocks): Grilled chicken and egg salad with fruit.

2 ounces (57 grams) (57 grams) grilled chicken, skinless

1 hard-boiled egg

Up to 2 heads of iceberg lettuce

1 cup (70 grams) (70 grams) raw mushrooms

1 cup (104 grams) raw cucumber, sliced 1 sliced red pepper

2 tablespoons avocado

1 teaspoon (5 ml) vinegar dressing

1 plum

Mid-Afternoon Snack (1 food block): Boiled egg, nuts and fruit.

1 hard-boiled egg

3 almonds 1/2 apple

Dinner (3 food blocks): Grilled salmon, lettuce and sweet potatoes.

4 oz (113 grams) (113 grams) salmon, grilled

2/3 cup (67 grams) of sweet potatoes, baked Up to 1 head of iceberg lettuce

1/4 cup (37 grams) (37 grams) raw tomato

1 cup (104 grams) (104 grams) raw cucumber, sliced 2 tablespoons avocado

1/3 teaspoon (3.3 ml) olive oil

Pre-Bedtime Snack (1 food block): Cottage cheese, nuts and fruit.

1/4 cup (56 grams) cottage cheese 6 peanuts

1/2 orange

A sample meal plan for women is similar to the plan for men, but has 11 food blocks instead of 14.

How to Prepare the Zone Diet & Tips

When following the Zone diet, you're urged to view food as a potent drug that has a powerful impact on your body and your health—more powerful "than any drug your doctor could ever prescribe," according to Dr. Sears. Every meal and snack should have the desired balance of macronutrients—protein, carbohydrates, and fat—that produce an appropriate and favorable hormonal response. First, you'll determine your total daily protein requirement. That amount of protein should be spread evenly throughout the day so that every meal you eat contains a roughly equal amount of protein. Every snack also should contain a smaller amount of protein.

According to Dr. Sears, everyone's daily protein requirement is unique. To calculate yours, first, calculate your percentage of body fat. Then, you use tables provided by Dr. Sears in his book to calculate total mass and lean body mass. Then, you'll balance your protein with carbohydrate foods—again, every meal and every snack should balance protein with carbohydrate, with a ratio of around one-third protein to two-thirds carbohydrate. Finally, you need to eat some fat at every meal. Fat in your diet helps to tell your body that you're full and don't need to eat any more food, and it serves as an important building block of the eicosanoid hormones that the Zone diet is attempting to promote. You need to know how much protein to eat when following the Zone diet since your protein allotment determines your carbohydrate and fat allotment. The key to determining your daily protein requirement is calculating your lean body mass and assessing how active you are. The Zone diet focuses heavily on keeping your body in "the Zone." Therefore, the timing of your daily food intake is critical to accomplish the diet's goals. Specifically, when following the Zone diet, you'll eat three meals a day: breakfast, lunch, and dinner. You'll also allow for two snacks.

Your meals will be evenly spaced throughout the day. Skipping meals is not recommended, nor is loading up at one meal and eating lightly at another. Just as you balance your food intake between protein, carbs, and fats, you'll balance it time-wise.

People who are following many other types of diets, such as a gluten-free diet, a vegetarian diet, or a diet that omits certain allergens such as nuts or cow's milk, also can follow the Zone diet with a few modifications:

The Zone diet doesn't require animal-based foods, so if you're a vegetarian or vegan, you can try the Zone diet. However, you should be aware that many plant-based staple foods, including grains and beans, are off-limits on the Zone diet due to their high starch content.

Since the Zone diet omits all grain-based foods (many of which contain gluten), it's easy to make it gluten-free. Therefore, people who have celiac disease or non-celiac gluten sensitivity may find that this diet fits in well with their goals and needs.

If you have diabetes, make sure to talk with your doctor before trying the Zone diet. The program is designed to help balance blood sugar, but people with diabetes could run into trouble by eliminating so many common foods at once.

Sample Shopping List

The Zone diet requires you to purchase a large amount of produce, including leafy greens. This might mean multiple shopping trips to buy fresh produce each week. Unless you have plenty of freezer space, if your lifestyle requires you to consume a lot of protein, you might need to make several trips for lean meats and fresh fish as well. Keep in mind, this is not a definitive shopping list, and if following the diet, you may find other foods that work best for you.

Lean meats (skinless chicken breasts, pork tenderloin) (skinless chicken breasts, pork tenderloin) Low-fat dairy (cottage cheese, yogurt) (cottage cheese, yogurt)

Fresh greens (kale, spinach, swiss chard) (kale, spinach, swiss chard) Fruit (apples, grapes, pears) (apples, grapes, pears)

Healthy fats (olive oil, nuts, natural peanut butter, avocado) (olive oil, nuts, natural peanut butter, avocado) Vegetables (zucchini, celery, cauliflower, broccoli) (zucchini, celery, cauliflower, broccoli)

Lean protein (eggs whites, tofu, protein powder) (eggs whites, tofu, protein powder)

Pros of the Zone Diet

General nutrition: The Zone diet generally follows nutritional guidance that calls for meals primarily carbohydrates, with a smaller amount of protein and a minimal amount of fat. Lean proteins are stressed, and the diet encourages you to consume lots of vegetables and fruit. Sugary drinks and other "junk food," such as candy and chips, are eliminated.

Flexibility: Since the diet allows such a wide variety of foods, it's pretty flexible. People who have other dietary restrictions should find it relatively simple to adapt. You will need to eat similarly sized meals three times per day, but many people already do this, so it won't be a significant change. Meal planning also isn't too tricky since many food combinations will work.

Healthy protein sources: The protein sources consumed on the Zone diet come from lean meats, tofu, egg whites, and low-fat dairy. Higher fat meats are consumed much less, leaving room in the diet for healthier unsaturated fats. Eating a higher-protein diet can prevent muscle loss, increase calorie burn, and keep you feeling full. And limiting saturated fats can improve cholesterol levels and overall heart health.

Cons of the Zone Diet

Difficult to sustain: Some people may find sticking to the Zone diet difficult because of the specific meal components. It is not easy to be sure you are eating the correct amount of protein, carbohydrates, and fats at each meal, especially if you are not at home. Some people may feel deprived due to the limited food choices, making a long-term commitment to this diet less likely.

Complicated tracking: Most diets call for tracking something—calories, carbs, or fat grams. The Zone diet is especially tricky since you'll need to count protein, fat, and carb grams all at once and make sure you consume the right quantities of each.

Unsubstantiated claims: Although the Zone diet is touted as one that can help you ward off serious chronic health conditions such as heart disease, diabetes, and cancer, people who already have been diagnosed with those conditions should talk to their doctors about whether the food restrictions in the diet are suitable for them.

Lacking fiber: The Zone diet eliminates many healthy food choices, such as whole- grain bread, cereal, pasta, beans and legumes, and some fruits. You may find it's challenging to get enough dietary fiber on this diet simply because it places so many good fiber choices off-limits. Fiber has been shown to help prevent and manage type 2 diabetes, cardiovascular disease, and some cancers. 3

Is the Zone Diet a Healthy Choice for You?

Although the Zone diet gets relatively good marks from nutritionists, it doesn't match up well with dietary recommendations from the U.S. Department of Agriculture (USDA) (USDA). The USDA's advice, outlined in the agency's MyPlate tool, calls for you to fill half of your plate with fruits and vegetables and the other half with protein and grains or starchy vegetables. Specific daily amounts are based on gender, physical activity, height, weight, and goals (such as a desire to gain, maintain, or lose weight) (such as a desire to gain, maintain, or lose weight). The protein amounts are similar between the USDA and the Zone diet, but the

Zone diet eliminates grain products. In terms of calorie intake, the Zone diet matches the USDA recommendations reasonably closely. Since the Zone diet is designed more to improve your health (with possible weight loss a bonus, not the goal), it doesn't focus on cutting calories substantially. According to Barry Sears, MD, "In the Zone, you'll enjoy optimal body function: freedom from hunger, greater energy, and physical performance, as well as improved mental focus and productivity." Since the diet consists of many healthy whole foods, this may well be true for you, but keep in mind that these claims have not been substantiated and this diet may not meet your specific needs. Speak to your doctor to see if the Zone diet is right for you.

How It Works

According to the diet, since carbohydrates and proteins are the determining nutrients for hormone activity, eating them in perfect combination is the most important rule. As with other low carbohydrate diets, the diet follows an average 40-30-30 ratio of macronutrient intake: 40 percent of caloric intake is complex carbohydrates, 30 percent of intake is protein and 30 percent of intake is fat. In order to achieve the "euphoria," there are favorable and unfavorable food lists from which to choose carbohydrate-, protein- and fat-containing foods. The program attempts to simplify the selection process and the counting of grams by using a "block" system. In general, the system identifies and recommends healthful sources of protein, fat and carbohydrate. For example, chicken breast and turkey breast are preferred over fattier meats such as bacon and pepperoni. Preferred carbohydrates include all vegetables and fruits that are not starchy, hence corn and potatoes are unfavorable choices.

According to the creator of the diet, following this simple eating pattern can alter your hormone levels and allow you to enter "the Zone," a physiological state that helps reduce levels of inflammation throughout the body. In addition to ramping up weight loss, maintaining this physiological state can also optimize cognitive health, slow signs of aging and boost the body's natural fat-burning abilities. In order to determine whether or not you're in "the Zone," Dr. Barry recommends testing your levels of three clinical markers, including:

Triglyceride (TG)/high-density lipoprotein (HDL) cholesterol ratio Arachidonic acid (AA)/eicosapentaenoic acid (EPA) ratio Hemoglobin A1C

If these three levels are within range, the body is said to be in "the Zone," meaning that you are able to reap the full rewards of the diet. The Zone Diet claims to optimize your hormones to allow your body to enter a state called "the Zone." This is where your body is optimized to control inflammation from your diet.

The alleged advantages of being in "the Zone" are: Losing extra body fat as fast as possible Maintaining wellness into older age Slowing down the rate of aging Performing better and thinking faster

Dr. Sears recommends testing three blood values to determine whether you are in "the Zone."

TG/HDL ratio

This is the ratio of "bad" fats known as triglycerides to "good" HDL cholesterol in your blood. A lower value means you have more good cholesterol, which is healthier. The Zone Diet recommends less than 1 as a good value, which is low. A high number for your TG/HDL ratio increases your risk of heart disease. Your ratio for TG/HDL must be tested by a health care professional, such as your doctor.

AA/EPA ratio

This is the ratio of omega-6 to omega-3 fats in your body. A lower value means you have more omega-3 fat in your blood, which is anti-inflammatory. The Zone Diet recommends a value between 1.5–3, which is low. A high number for your AA/EPA ratio is linked with a higher risk of depression, obesity and other chronic diseases. You can test your ratio for AA/EPA at home with a kit purchased on the Zone Diet website.

HbA1c, also known as glycated hemoglobin

This is a marker of your average blood sugar levels over the preceding three months. A lower value means you have less sugar in your blood. The Zone Diet recommends a value of less than 5 percent , which is low. A higher HbA1c is linked to a higher risk of diabetes. Your HbA1c must be tested by a health care professional, such as your doctor.

Supplements recommended

The Zone Diet recommends that you take omega-3 supplements, such as fish oil, to maximize health benefits. They decrease the "bad" LDL cholesterol in your body, and may reduce your risk of other chronic health diseases. The Zone Diet also recommends taking polyphenol supplements, which are molecules found in plants that have antioxidant properties. The evidence behind polyphenols is mixed, and while it may have health benefits such as lowering the risk of heart disease, it also has risks such as lowering iron absorption. The Zone Diet purports to reduce inflammation in the body. You can find out if you're in "the Zone" by taking a blood test. Omega-3 fatty acids and polyphenols are recommended supplements.

The Zone Diet has a lot of advantages.

There are a lot of advantages to sticking to the Zone Diet. The Zone Diet, unlike other diets, does not impose strict dietary restrictions. It does, however, advise against unhealthy choices like added sugar and processed foods. For people who struggle with food restrictions, this may make the Zone Diet more appealing than other diets. The Zone Diet's food recommendations are very similar to those of the Mediterranean Diet. Evidence supports the Mediterranean Diet as one of the best for long-term health. Because there are two ways to follow the Zone Diet, you have a lot of flexibility. The Zone Food Block method can also aid fat loss by limiting the number of calories consumed each day. Controlling your calorie intake is well known to aid weight loss.

You can find out how many calories you need to consume per day to maintain and lose weight here. The benefits of the Zone Diet are numerous, and they are linked to the diet's favorable foods. It's adaptable and can help you lose weight by limiting your calorie intake.

Advantages to Your Health

The Zone Diet promotes a wide variety of healthy foods and does not impose any strict restrictions on which ingredients should be avoided or restricted. As a result, it may be a good choice for dieters looking for variety and flexibility. It also has a lot in common with the Mediterranean diet, which consists of fruits, vegetables, nuts, seeds, and whole grains. The Mediterranean diet has been shown to protect against heart disease, cancer, diabetes, and neurodegenerative disorders like Alzheimer's disease in studies. While more research is needed, a similar diet pattern, such as the Zone Diet, could provide similar health benefits. Because the diet emphasizes low-glycemic, minimally processed foods, it may also improve the overall quality of your diet. In fact, studies show that eating a low-glycemic diet can improve blood sugar control and the body's ability to use insulin effectively.

Furthermore, other studies have linked eating fewer processed foods to a lower risk of weight gain. Many people associate the Zone Diet with CrossFit, a high-intensity interval training workout. The Zone Diet, which is high in protein, may aid tissue repair and muscle growth, giving your workout a boost. However, studies on the impact of diet on athletic performance have yielded mixed results. As a result, more research is needed to determine how the Zone Diet affects exercise.

Risks, Side Effects, and Negative Consequences

Although the Zone Diet may have some advantages, it also has some drawbacks.

Also think about it. To begin with, there is little to no research to back up the diet's premise. "A review of the literature suggests that there are scientific contradictions in the Zone Diet hypothesis that cast unquestionable doubt on its potential efficacy," according to a study published in the Journal of the American College of Nutrition. Some people may find the diet difficult to stick to over time. To maintain the macronutrient ratio recommended by the diet, the block method, in particular, may necessitate meticulous food tracking and measurement. The hand-eye method is a good alternative for those looking for a more straightforward method, but it may not be as accurate. Furthermore, some research suggests that the Zone Diet may not be the best option for everyone in terms of athletic performance.

Athletes who followed the diet for one week experienced a significant drop in endurance and became exhausted much more quickly, according to one study. "This is not a nutritional strategy that athletes should use until more research has been conducted," the study's authors write. The Zone Diet has several advantages, but it also has some drawbacks.

To begin with, the Zone Diet makes a number of bold health claims that are based on the diet's theory. However, there is little evidence that the theory achieves the claimed outcomes. The Zone Diet, for example, claims to improve performance. However, a study of athletes who followed the diet discovered that, while they lost weight, they also lost endurance and became exhausted more quickly than others. Another claim made by the diet is that it can help you reach "the Zone" by reducing diet-induced inflammation. According to the Zone Diet, your body will be in "the Zone" once your blood values reach their goals.

Although some research suggests that the diet can improve blood pressure, more research is needed before researchers can conclude that it significantly reduces inflammation in the body. There's also little evidence that the Zone Diet's 40 percent carb, 30 percent protein, and 30 percent fat ratio is the best for fat loss and overall health. Another study compared the effects of a Zone-style diet with 40% carbs, 30% protein, and 30% fat to the effects of a diet with 60% carbs, 15% protein, and 25% fat. People who followed a Zone-based diet lost more weight, according to the research. That difference, however, could be due to a higher protein intake. Surprisingly, there were no significant differences in blood sugar, fat, or cholesterol levels between the two groups, according to the study. This contradicts the Zone Diet's claims, and it's possible that the improved blood values seen in other studies are due to omega-3 and polyphenol supplementation rather than dietary benefits. The Zone Diet boasts a slew of health benefits. However, there isn't enough proof to back them up.

Should you give the Zone Diet a shot?

Finally, pick a diet that best fits your lifestyle. If you want a diet that has similar food options to the Mediterranean Diet but with clear guidelines to follow, the Zone Diet might be right for you. However, the diet's health claims should be taken with a grain of salt. Although the diet's theory may be linked to improved health outcomes, there is insufficient evidence to claim that it will reduce your risk of chronic disease, slow down aging, improve physical performance, or help you think faster.

If you want to try to develop healthy eating habits, the Zone Diet may be able to assist you in getting started and practicing portion control. However, regardless of the name of the diet, what matters in the long run is that you base your diet on whole, unprocessed foods.

Is the Zone Diet going to help you lose weight?

Probably. Any calorie-restricted diet will aid weight loss. Zone appears to be moderately effective for weight loss, based on limited research. However, the 40-30-30 carbohydrate-protein-fat ratio isn't a magic bullet, and some scientific evidence questions its effectiveness.

A systematic review published in April 2020 looked at research on 14 popular diets to see how well they lost weight and reduced heart risk factors. More than 120 studies on nearly 22,000 overweight or obese participants were included in the review, which was published in the journal BMJ. When compared to a standard diet, Zone was one of the top three popular diets for weight loss and blood pressure control. At the six-month mark, zone participants had lost an average of 9 pounds.

In a 2007 study published in the Journal of the American Medical Association, researchers divided 300 overweight or obese women into four groups and assigned them to one of four diets: low-carb (Atkins), low-fat (Ornish), low-saturated-fat/moderate-carb (LEARN), and roughly equal parts protein, fat, and carb (LEARN). Zone dieters lost about 6 pounds after two months, about the same as the other groups – with the exception of the Atkins group, which lost 9.5 pounds. After a year, the Zone group lost an average of 3.5 pounds, which was less than the other groups. The Atkins group lost 10 pounds, while the LEARN group lost 6 pounds and the Ornish group lost 5.

According to findings published in the Journal of the American Medical Association in 2005, weight loss was modest for all groups in a study of 160 people assigned to the Zone, Atkins, Weight Watchers, or Ornish diet. After a year, Zone dieters had lost an average of 7 pounds, compared to 7.3 pounds for the Ornish group, 6.6 pounds for Weight Watchers, and 4.6 pounds for Atkins, and Zone (and Weight Watchers) dieters had dropped out at a lower rate (around 35 percent) than Atkins and Ornish dieters. Around 25% of dieters in all groups had lost more than 5% of their starting weight, and 10% had lost more than 10%. This is critical because if you're overweight, losing just 5 to 10% of your current weight can help you avoid certain diseases.

Researchers looked at existing research on the Atkins, South Beach, Weight Watchers, and Zone diets to see which was the most effective, according to a study published in Circulation: Cardiovascular Quality and Outcomes in November 2014. Their findings suggested that none of the four diet plans resulted in significant weight loss, and that none of them were significantly better than the others at keeping weight off for a year or longer.

Each of the four diet plans helped dieters lose roughly the same amount of weight in the short term: about 5% of their initial body weight. Those on the Atkins or Weight Watchers plans, however, regained some of the weight they had lost after two years. Because the diets produce similar results, the researchers concluded that dieters should pick the one that best fits their lifestyle – for example, Weight Watchers uses a group-based, behavior-modification approach, while Atkins focuses on carbohydrate restriction.

How easy is it to stick to the Zone Diet?

Keeping track of the right proportions of carbs, protein, and healthy fat in each meal necessitates forethought. Zone's strict eating schedule – breakfast within one hour of waking up, followed by snacks and meals every five hours – may be too much for some dieters.

Recipes are available, but adhering to the 40-30-30 rule may take some time. It is possible to eat out on a regular basis. The firm's online and printed resources could be useful.

You can eat out as long as you avoid the bread basket, order a low-fat protein entree, and avoid starches and grains. Examine the size of your entree once it arrives. Plan to take some home if it's larger than your palm. Zone pasta, bars, and cereals are designed to help you stick to the diet and can help suppress your appetite, but they're not required.

Zonediet.com offers a free online membership that includes a body fat calculator, monthly newsletters, recipes, and health podcasts and videocasts. For answers to specific questions and emotional support, you can speak live with a Zone customer service representative during business hours on weekdays. Diet education and training is ongoing for representatives. As needed, the staff wellness director and dietitian can offer more advanced assistance. Support is also available via email and the Zone Facebook page.

On this diet, hunger shouldn't be an issue. The Zone diet necessitates strategic snacking – you won't go more than five hours without eating. According to Sears, this will keep your blood sugar stable and prevent hunger pangs.

On the Zone diet, you don't have to give up flavor. From blueberry pancakes to pork medallions, there's something for everyone. Cheese, wine, and peanuts are some of the snacks available. You also don't have to give up your personal favorites. It's fine to indulge once in a while as long as you get back on track the next day.

On the Zone Diet, how much exercise should you do?

The Zone diet encourages but does not require exercise. Sears claims that exercise is more important for weight maintenance than for weight loss, a claim that the mainstream medical community may not agree with. Most experts recommend getting at least 2.5 hours of moderate-intensity activity (like brisk walking) per week, along with a couple days of muscle-strengthening activities, whether for general health or weight loss. Whatever diet you follow, the more you move, the faster you'll lose weight – and the lower your risk of diabetes, heart disease, and other chronic diseases.

Finally, some advice

Chapter Fourteen

What is the Zone Diet, exactly? The Zone Diet is a well-known eating plan that aims to reduce inflammation and improve overall health.

Despite their similar names, the Zone Diet is unrelated to the blue zone diet or the keto zone diet, both of which are health-promoting eating plans.

The Zone Diet consists of roughly 40% carbohydrates, 30% protein, and 30% fat, which can be calculated using the hand-eye or block method.

Despite the fact that no foods are strictly forbidden on the diet, a typical meal plan should consist primarily of lean proteins, low-glycemic carbohydrates, and monounsaturated fats. The diet is similar to the Mediterranean diet, which has been shown to protect against disease, and encourages a variety of healthy foods. Another benefit of the Zone Diet could be that it encourages higher protein intake and low-glycemic foods.

On the other hand, there is little evidence to back up the Zone Diet's premise. It may also be difficult to follow in the long run, and athletes may not find it to be a good choice.

As a result, while the Zone Diet may be a useful tool for establishing healthy habits, eating a variety of healthy, minimally processed foods can be equally effective in promoting long-term health.

Recipes for Zone Diet Recipe Summary for Diet Soup

20-minute prep

30 minutes in the oven

50 minutes total

8 people

8 servings (approximately).

Ingredients

Section 2:

Chapter Fifteen

Step 1: Follow the directions

1 medium head cabbage, chopped 1 onion, chopped\s3 big carrots, chopped 3 stalks celery, chopped 3 tomatoes, chopped\s16 ounces frozen green beans\s2 (1 ounce) packets dry onion soup mix 6 cups water

Combine water, soup mix, and vegetables in a large stock pot. Bring to a boil. Reduce heat, and simmer until the veggies are soft.

Nutrition Facts\sPer Serving: 94 calories; protein 3.6g; carbs 21g; fat 0.5g; sodium 672.9mg. Chocolate Chip Cookies for Special Diets

Recipe Summary Prep: 15 mins

Cook: 12 minutes

Additional: 23 mins

50 minutes total

Servings: 48

Yield: 4 dozen

Ingredients

½ cup butter, softened

¾ cup granulated artificial sweetener 2 tablespoons water\s½ teaspoon vanilla extract 1 egg, beaten

1 ⅛ cups all-purpose flour

½ teaspoon baking soda

½ teaspoon salt

½ cup semisweet chocolate chips

½ cup chopped pecans

Directions Step 1

Preheat oven to 375 degrees F (190 degrees C) (190 degrees C).

Step 2

In a medium bowl, cream together the butter and sugar substitute. Mix in water, vanilla, and egg. Sift together the flour, baking soda, and salt; stir into the creamed mixture. Mix in the chocolate chips and pecans. Drop cookies by heaping teaspoonfuls onto a cookie sheet.

Step 3

Bake in the preheated oven for 10 to 12 minutes. Remove from cookie sheets to cool on wire racks. These cookies freeze well.

Nutrition Facts

Per Serving: 60 calories; protein 4.2g; carbohydrates 3.5g; fat 3.4g; cholesterol 9mg; sodium 53.8mg.

Kitchen Sink Soup

Recipe Summary 20-minute prep

30 minutes in the oven

50 minutes total

Servings: 10

Yield: 10 servings

Ingredients

10 cups chicken broth 2 potatoes, cubed\s2 carrots, sliced\s2 stalks celery, diced\s5 fresh mushrooms, sliced\s1 green bell pepper, chopped 1 fresh broccoli, chopped\s4 cups cauliflower florets 1 parsnip, sliced\s1 onion, chopped 1 cup green peas

1 cup cut green beans, drained 1 cup wax beans, drained\s½ cup cooked chickpeas

½ cup cooked navy beans salt and pepper to taste

1 teaspoon dried parsley

Directions Step 1

In a large stockpot, combine all the ingredients and cook over medium heat partially covered for about 30 minutes or until all the vegetables are tender. Serve hot with buttered biscuits.

Nutrition Facts

Per Serving: 160 calories; protein 10.3g; carbohydrates 26.3g; fat 1.9g; sodium 1008.1mg.

Gluten-Free Chocolate Chip Cookies\sRecipe Summary Prep: 15 mins

Cook: 10 mins

Additional: 10 mins

Total: 35 mins

Servings: 24

Yield: 2 dozen

Ingredients

½ cup coconut palm sugar

¼ cup extra-virgin coconut oil, at room temperature

½ teaspoon baking soda Himalayan pink salt to taste 2 cups almond flour

2 eggs

1 tablespoon vanilla extract

1 cup chocolate chips (such as Ghirardelli®)

Directions Step 1

Preheat oven to 350 degrees F (175 degrees C). Lightly grease a baking sheet.

Step 2

Combine coconut sugar, coconut oil, baking soda, and salt in a large bowl; beat with a handheld electric mixer until smooth. Add almond flour, eggs, and vanilla extract. Beat dough at medium speed, scraping the bottom and sides of the bowl, until well mixed, about 1 minute.

Step 3

Fold chocolate chips into the dough. Grease your palms lightly with coconut oil; drop tablespoonfuls of dough onto the baking sheet.

Step 4

Bake in the preheated oven until golden brown, 10 to 12 minutes. Let cool on the baking sheet, about 10 minutes.

Nutrition Facts

Per Serving: 139 calories; protein 3g; carbohydrates 11.2g; fat 9.9g; cholesterol 15.5mg; sodium 36.2mg.

Low-Carb Pancakes with Coconut Flour Recipe Summary Prep: 10 mins

Cook: 20 mins

Total: 30 mins

Servings: 6

Yield: 6 pancakes

Ingredients

1 teaspoon butter, or as needed 4 eggs

½ cup Greek yogurt

¼ cup water ¼ cup coconut flour

2 tablespoons coconut oil, melted 1 tablespoon flaxseed meal

2 teaspoons vanilla extract

2 teaspoons gluten-free baking powder 2 teaspoons ground cinnamon

½ teaspoon salt ½ teaspoon stevia powder

Directions Step 1

Heat a cast iron skillet over medium-low heat and grease with butter.

Step 2

Whisk eggs, yogurt, water, coconut flour, coconut oil, flaxseed meal, vanilla extract, baking powder, cinnamon, salt, and stevia together in a large bowl.

Step 3

Drop batter into the hot skillet using a 1/3 cup measuring cup. Cook until bubbles form and the pancakes are firm enough to flip, 4 to 5 minutes. Be sure to cook them on low enough heat that the outside doesn't burn before the inside is done. Flip and cook until browned on the other side and done in the middle, 2 to 3 minutes. Repeat with remaining batter.

Nutrition Facts

Per Serving: 151 calories; protein 6.2g; carbohydrates 6.5g; fat 11.3g; cholesterol 129.5mg; sodium 419.5mg.

Aunt Rocky's Fluffy LCHF Pancakes (Low Carb, Grain Free, Gluten Free, Low Glycemic) Recipe Summary Prep: 10 mins

Cook: 3 mins

Total: 13 mins

Servings: 12

Yield: 12 pancakes

Ingredients

½ cup coconut flour

1 ½ tablespoons erythritol 1 tablespoon oat fiber (such as LifeSource Foods®)

½ teaspoon gluten-free baking powder (such as Rumford®)

¼ teaspoon xanthan gum 1 pinch salt

1 teaspoon oil, or as desired 5 large eggs

½ cup butter, melted 3 tablespoons water

3 tablespoons heavy whipping cream

1 teaspoon cider vinegar (such as Bragg®)

1 teaspoon vanilla extract

Directions Step 1

Whisk coconut flour, erythritol, oat fiber, baking powder, xanthan gum, and salt together in a bowl, breaking up any lumps in the coconut flour.

Step 2

Preheat a griddle or pan over medium-low heat and lightly oil the surface.

Step 3

Mix eggs, butter, water, cream, vinegar, and vanilla extract into the bowl with the coconut flour mixture. Stir well to combine; batter will be thicker than regular pancake batter.

Step 4

Scoop 1/4 cup batter at a time onto the preheated griddle, leaving space between each pancake and smoothing the tops slightly. Cook until bubbles form, edges begin to dry, and the bottom is browned, 2 to 5 minutes. Flip pancakes carefully using a thin spatula; continue cooking until firm and browned on the second side, about 1 minute more.

Cook's Notes:

If you can't get oat fiber, you can try substituting psyllium husk powder. The texture won't be quite the same, but the recipe will work.

You can use the same amount of glucomannan in place of xanthan gum.

If batter gets too thick to scoop, add 1 tablespoon of water and whisk again.

Get the pans out before you begin. These pancakes are cooked on a lower heat to keep them from burning, so they'll take longer than regular pancakes. You'll get 3 pancakes per 12" round pan, and 4 pancakes in a square pan. If you have the pans and the stove space, it will go quicker using 2 pans at one time.

Nutrition Facts

Per Serving: 133 calories; protein 3.5g; carbohydrates 6.5g; fat 11.4g; cholesterol 100.4mg; sodium 120.1mg.

Juicy Slow Cooker Chicken Breast For Any Diet

Recipe Summary Prep: 10 mins

Cook: 6 hrs

Total: 6 hrs 10 mins

Servings: 4

Yield: 4 servings

Ingredients

1 pound skinless, boneless chicken breast halves 1 (14.5 ounce) can petite diced tomatoes

¼ onion, chopped (Optional)

1 teaspoon Italian seasoning (Optional) 1 clove garlic, minced (Optional)

Directions Step 1

Arrange chicken in a slow cooker. Pour tomatoes over chicken; add onion, Italian seasoning, and garlic.

Step 2

Cook on Low for 6 to 8 hours.

Cook's Note:

You can use any type of herb in place of the Italian seasoning.

Nutrition Facts

Per Serving: 144 calories; protein 23.1g; carbohydrates 5.2g; fat 2.4g; cholesterol 58.5mg; sodium 208mg.

Lemon Garlic Chicken Breasts Recipe Summary Prep: 10 mins

Cook: 25 mins

Total: 35 mins

Servings: 4

Yield: 4 servings

Ingredients

cooking spray

1 clove garlic, minced

4 skinless, boneless chicken breast halves salt and ground black pepper to taste

¾ cup chicken broth

1 tablespoon lemon juice

Directions Step 1

Lightly spray a nonstick skillet with cooking spray and place over low heat; cook and stir garlic until fragrant and lightly browned, 2 to 3 minutes.

Step 2

Season chicken with salt and pepper and place in skillet with garlic; cook over medium heat until browned on both sides, 10 to 12 minutes. Add chicken broth and lemon juice; bring to a boil. Reduce heat to medium-low, cover skillet, and simmer until chicken is no longer pink in the center, 10 to 15 minutes. An instant-read thermometer inserted into the center should read at least 165 degrees F (74 degrees C).

Step 3

Transfer chicken to a serving dish, reserving liquid in skillet. Continue simmering liquid until slightly reduced, about 3 minutes. Pour liquid over chicken.

Nutrition Facts

Per Serving: 131 calories; protein 23.8g; carbohydrates 0.8g; fat 2.9g; cholesterol 65.5mg; sodium 275.2mg.

Pollo Guisado Recipe Summary Prep: 15 mins

Cook: 1 hr 35 mins

Total: 1 hr 50 mins

8 people

8 servings (approximately).

Ingredients

2 tablespoons olive oil 1 whole chicken, cut up salt and ground black pepper to taste 1 medium onion, chopped 4 cloves garlic,

minced ½ cup sofrito 2 potatoes, peeled and cubed 2 cups chicken broth

1 (8 ounce) can tomato sauce

1 (1.41 ounce) package sazon seasoning

½ teaspoon ground cumin 1 bay leaf

2 tablespoons cold water 1 tablespoon cornstarch

Directions Step 1

Heat olive oil over medium-high heat in a Dutch oven. Season chicken with salt and pepper and add to the hot pot to brown, 6 to 7 minutes per side. Transfer chicken a bowl and cover with an aluminum foil tent.

Step 2

Reduce heat to medium; add onion to the pot and saute until translucent, about 5 minutes. Add garlic and cook for 1 minute. Stir in sofrito and cook for 2 to 3 minutes. Add potatoes, chicken broth, tomato sauce, sazon, cumin, and bay leaf; bring to a boil. Return chicken to the pot. Cover and cook for 1 hour. Remove chicken.

Step 3

Mix water and cornstarch together in a small bowl; stir into simmering mixture until nicely thickened. Place chicken back into the pot and continue to cook about 10 minutes more.

Nutrition Facts

Per Serving: 278 calories; protein 18.7g; carbohydrates 14.3g; fat 16g; cholesterol 47.6mg; sodium 1339.4mg.

Balsamic Marinated Chicken Breasts Recipe Summary Prep: 15 mins

Cook: 40 mins

Additional: 30 mins

Total: 1 hr 25 mins

Servings: 4

Yield: 4 chicken breasts

Ingredients

¾ cup balsamic vinegar

½ cup water

1 teaspoon dried minced onion

½ teaspoon crushed red pepper flakes

½ teaspoon dried minced garlic

¼ teaspoon salt ¼ teaspoon ground black pepper

¼ teaspoon paprika

¼ teaspoon crushed dried rosemary

¼ teaspoon dried parsley flakes

¼ teaspoon chili powder

⅛ teaspoon dried oregano

4 (6 ounce) skinless, boneless chicken breast halves

Step 1: Follow the directions

Whisk together the balsamic vinegar, water, onion, red pepper flakes, garlic, salt, pepper, paprika, rosemary, parsley, chili powder, and oregano in a bowl, and pour into a resealable plastic bag. Add the chicken breasts, coat with the marinade, squeeze out excess air, and seal the bag. Marinate in the refrigerator 30 minutes to overnight.

Step 2

Preheat oven to 400 degrees F (200 degrees C). Line a baking sheet with aluminum foil, or lightly grease a broiler pan. Remove the chicken breasts from the marinade, and shake off excess. Discard the remaining marinade, and place the chicken breasts onto the baking sheet.

Step 3

Bake in the preheated oven until the chicken breasts are golden brown and no longer pink in the center, 30 to 40 minutes. An instant-read thermometer inserted into the center should reach 165 degrees F (74 degrees C).

Nutrition Facts

Per Serving: 222 calories; protein 35.7g; carbohydrates 8g; fat 4.3g; cholesterol 96.9mg; sodium 244.3mg.

Eggless Pasta Recipe Summary Servings: 4 Yield: 4 cups of noodles

Ingredients

2 cups semolina flour ½ teaspoon salt

½ cup warm water

Directions Step 1

In a large bowl, mix flour and salt. Add warm water and stir to make a stiff dough. Increase water if dough seems too dry.

Step 2

Pat the dough into a ball and turn out onto a lightly floured surface. Knead for 10 to 15 minutes. Cover. Let dough rest for 20 minutes.

Step 3

Roll out dough using rolling pin or pasta machine. Work with a 1/4 of the dough at one time. Keep the rest covered, to prevent from drying out. Roll by hand to 1/16 of an inch thick. By machine, stop at the third to last setting.

Step 4

Cut pasta into desired shapes.

Step 5

Cook fresh noodles in boiling salted water for 3 to 5 minutes. Drain.

Nutrition Facts Per Serving: 301 calories; protein 10.6g; carbohydrates 60.8g; fat 0.9g; sodium 292.4mg. Spelt Noodles Recipe Summary Servings: 2 Yield: 2 servings

Ingredients

1 cup white spelt flour 1 egg

1 tablespoon vegetable oil

3 tablespoons water as needed

Directions Step 1 (Preferred) Process all ingredients in a food processor until they form a ball that rides on the blades.

Step 2

You can also let a bread machine knead the ingredients for about 5 minutes. (I've never tried this,

but have heard it works well.)

Step 3

Pasta can be rolled and cut in a regular (manual, hand-crank) pasta maker by passing it through repeatedly smaller (i.e., higher number) settings until nearly paper thin, and then run through the cutting blades. I am told it does not do so well in an automatic pasta maker.

Nutrition Facts

Per Serving: 297 calories; protein 11.1g; carbohydrates 42.2g; fat 10.4g; cholesterol 93mg; sodium 37.7mg.

Tequila-Lime Chicken Recipe Summary Prep: 10 mins

Cook: 35 mins

Additional: 1 hr

Total: 1 hr 45 mins

Servings: 4

Yield: 4 servings

Ingredients

3 skinless, boneless chicken breasts

½ cup tequila

1 lime, zested and juiced ¼ teaspoon garlic powder, divided ¼ teaspoon chili powder, divided

3 ounces shredded Mexican-style cheese blend

Directions Step 1

Arrange chicken breasts in a baking dish; add tequila and juice of 1/2 a lime. Sprinkle 1/2 of the lime zest, 1/2 of the garlic powder, and 1/2 of the chili powder over the chicken. Cover dish with plastic wrap and marinate in the refrigerator for 30 minutes.

Step 2

Turn chicken breasts; sprinkle remaining lime juice, lime zest, garlic powder, and chili powder on top. Cover again and marinate in the refrigerator for another 30 minutes.

Step 3

Preheat the oven to 425 degrees F (220 degrees C). Uncover baking dish and discard tequila-lime marinade.

Step 4

Bake chicken in the preheated oven for 25 minutes. Sprinkle Mexican-style cheese over the chicken and continue to bake until the chicken is no longer pink in the center and the juices run clear, about 10 minutes more. An instant-read thermometer inserted into the center should read at least 165 degrees F (74 degrees C).

Editor's Note:

Nutrition data for this recipe includes the full amount of marinade ingredients. The actual amount of marinade consumed will vary.

Nutrition Facts

Per Serving: 244 calories; protein 22.5g; carbohydrates 1.7g; fat 8.8g; cholesterol 68.8mg; sodium 207mg.

Chocolate-y Iced Mocha Recipe Summary Prep: 5 mins

Cook: 1 min

Total: 6 mins

Servings: 1

Yield: 1 serving

Ingredients

1 ¼ cups cold coffee, divided 1 envelope low-calorie hot cocoa mix ice cubes, or as needed

Chapter Sixteen

Step 1: Follow the directions

½ cup unsweetened almond milk

2 tablespoons sugar-free chocolate syrup, or more to taste

Heat 1/4 cup coffee in microwave in a mug until warmed, about 30 seconds. Stir cocoa mix into the coffee until dissolved.

Step 2

Fill a large glass with ice cubes. Pour 1 cup cold coffee and almond milk over the ice cubes; stir the cocoa mixture and chocolate syrup into the coffee and almond milk.

Nutrition Facts

Per Serving: 105 calories; protein 5.2g; carbohydrates 16.7g; fat 1.8g; cholesterol 2.9mg; sodium 255.3mg.

Sugar-Free Cream Cheese Frosting Recipe Summary Prep: 5 mins

Total: 5 mins

Servings: 12

Yield: 12 servings

Ingredients

1 (8 ounce) package reduced-fat cream cheese, softened ½ cup granular sucrolose sweetener (such as Splenda®), or more to taste 1 (8 ounce) container frozen whipped topping, thawed 1 teaspoon vanilla extract

Directions Step 1

Beat cream cheese and sucralose sweetener together in a bowl using an electric mixer until smooth and creamy; stir in whipped topping and vanilla extract until smooth.

Nutrition Facts

Per Serving: 104 calories; protein 2.2g; carbohydrates 5.7g; fat 8.1g; cholesterol 10.6mg; sodium 60.7mg.

Skinny Chocolate Mocha Shake Recipe Summary Prep: 5 mins

Additional: 2 hrs

Total: 2 hrs 5 mins

Servings: 1

Yield: 1 serving

Ingredients

1 cup Gevalia® Cold Brew Concentrate - House Blend 1 envelope sugar free instant cocoa mix

¼ cup hot water ¼ cup soy milk

2 tablespoons sugar free chocolate syrup

1 packet sugar substitute (such as Truvia®) (Optional)

Directions Step 1

Place cold brew concentrate in ice cube tray(s); place in freezer until frozen solid, 2 to 4 hours.

Step 2

Dissolve hot cocoa mix in hot water.

Step 3

Place coffee cubes in a blender. Add cocoa mixture, soy milk, chocolate syrup, and sweetener. Blend until icy and frothy, 1 or 2 minutes.

Cook's Note:

Top with fat free whip cream if desired.

Editor's Note:

This recipe was developed by this Allrecipes Allstar as part of a campaign sponsored by Gevalia.

Nutrition Facts

Per Serving: 123 calories; protein 6.3g; carbohydrates 21g; fat 1.5g; cholesterol 2.9mg; sodium 242.5mg.

Creamy Cream Cheese Frosting Recipe Summary Prep: 10 mins

Total: 10 mins

Servings: 12

Yield: 1 frosting for 1 cake

Ingredients

1 (3 ounce) package cream cheese 1 ¾ cups confectioners' sugar

1 (8 ounce) container frozen whipped topping, thawed

Directions Step 1

In a large bowl, beat cream cheese and sugar until smooth. Fold in whipped topping.

Nutrition Facts

Per Serving: 155 calories; protein 0.8g; carbohydrates 22.7g; fat 7.2g; cholesterol 7.8mg; sodium 25.8mg.

Orange Mocha Recipe Summary Prep: 5 mins

Total: 5 mins

Servings: 1

Yield: 1 servings

Ingredients

1 cup brewed coffee

2 tablespoons orange juice 2 tablespoons milk 1 tablespoon white sugar

1 tablespoon unsweetened cocoa powder

Directions Step 1 Stir coffee, orange juice, milk, sugar, and cocoa powder together in a mug until the sugar and cocoa dissolve.

Nutrition Facts

Per Serving: 92 calories; protein 2.6g; carbohydrates 20.1g; fat 1.5g; cholesterol 2.4mg; sodium 18.7mg.

Keto-Friendly Bread Recipe Summary Prep: 15 mins

Cook: 35 mins

Additional: 10 mins

Total: 1 hr

8 people

8 servings (approximately).

Ingredients

cooking spray

6 eggs, separated ¼ teaspoon cream of tartar 6 tablespoons coconut flour 6 tablespoons almond flour

Chapter Seventeen

Step 1: Follow the directions

2 tablespoons arrowroot powder

1 teaspoon gluten-free baking powder

½ teaspoon kosher salt

¼ cup coconut oil, melted and cooled 1 tablespoon honey

Preheat the oven to 350 degrees F (175 degrees C). Spray a 4x8-inch loaf pan with cooking spray.

Step 2

Beat egg whites in a glass, metal, or ceramic bowl until foamy. Gradually add cream of tartar, continuing to beat until soft peaks form. Set aside.

Step 3

Combine coconut flour, almond flour, arrowroot powder, baking powder, and salt in a bowl and mix well.

Step 4

Beat egg yolks using an electric mixer in a bowl until thick. Add coconut oil and honey; mix well. Add flour mixture and stir until well combined. Fold in 1/4 of the beaten egg whites until incorporated. Add 1/2 the remaining egg whites and gently fold until only small amounts of egg whites are visible. Repeat with remaining egg whites. Pour mixture into prepared loaf pan and smooth the top.

Step 5

Bake in the preheated oven until nicely golden brown on top, about 35 minutes. Remove from oven, set on a wire rack, and let cool for 10 minutes. Run a knife around the sides, tip out bread onto a rack, and let cool completely.

Cook's Note:

The bread can be flavored in any way you like, for example, with a little artificial sweetener and almond, orange, or lemon extract for a breakfast or dessert treat, or herbs for a savory side.

Nutrition Facts

Per Serving: 181 calories; protein 6.3g; carbohydrates 9.8g; fat 13.7g; cholesterol 122.8mg; sodium 227.3mg.

Whole Wheat Oatmeal Strawberry Blueberry Muffins Recipe Summary 20-minute prep

Cook:

18 mins

Total:

38 mins

Servings:

12

Yield:

12 servings

Ingredients

1 cup whole wheat flour 1 cup oats

½ cup white sugar

2 teaspoons baking powder

½ teaspoon baking soda

½ teaspoon salt 1 cup milk

¼ cup vegetable oil 1 egg

1 teaspoon vanilla extract 2 cups diced strawberries 1 cup fresh blueberries

Step 1: Follow the directions

Preheat oven to 425 degrees F (220 degrees C). Grease muffin cups or line with paper muffin liners.

Step 2

Mix flour, oats, sugar, baking powder, baking soda, and salt together in a bowl. Combine milk, vegetable oil, egg, and vanilla extract in a separate bowl.

Step 3

Stir milk mixture into flour mixture until batter is combined. Fold in strawberries and blueberries. Spoon batter into prepared muffin pan until full.

Step 4

Bake in preheated oven until a toothpick inserted into the center comes out clean, 18 to 22 minutes.

Nutrition Facts

Per Serving: 164 calories; protein 3.7g; carbohydrates 25.1g; fat 6.1g; cholesterol 15.3mg; sodium 245.4mg.

Spiced Zucchini Carrot Muffins Recipe Summary Prep: 25 mins

Cook: 20 mins

Total: 45 mins

Servings: 21

Yield: 21 muffins

Ingredients

1 cup butter

1 cup white sugar 3 eggs

2 cups grated zucchini 1 cup grated carrots

3 teaspoons vanilla extract

Chapter Eighteen

Step 1: Follow the directions

3 cups all-purpose flour

2 teaspoons ground nutmeg

2 teaspoons ground cinnamon 1 teaspoon salt 1 teaspoon baking soda

¼ teaspoon baking powder

½ cup raisins (Optional)

½ cup chopped walnuts (Optional)

Preheat the oven to 350 degrees F (175 degrees C). Grease two 12-cup muffin tins or line cups with paper liners.

Step 2

Combine butter, sugar, and eggs in a large bowl; beat with an electric mixer until creamy. Beat in zucchini, carrots, and vanilla extract.

Step 3

Combine flour, nutmeg, cinnamon, salt, baking soda, and baking powder in a separate bowl. Mix into the creamed butter mixture. Stir in raisins and walnuts. Pour batter into the greased muffin cups.

Step 4

Bake in the preheated oven until a toothpick inserted into the center comes out clean, about 17 minutes.

Substitute pumpkin pie spice for the nutmeg if preferred.

Nutrition Facts

Per Serving: 227 calories; protein 3.6g; carbohydrates 28g; fat 11.6g; cholesterol 49.8mg; sodium 254.4mg.

Chapter Nineteen

So, in terms of fat loss, this diet is very good so long as you are willing to put in the effort required. If you are looking for a simple plan however, where you can eat out easily and don't always need to be watching the clock, this likely isn't a good choice. With regards to muscle building on the other hand, it can definitely be used and again is probably preferable over keto for muscle building as there are more carbohydrates allowed.

Generally speaking, carbohydrates tend to be quite anabolic, more so than fat due to their effect on insulin so this diet caters to that more effectively. The nice thing about this diet with respect to that issue also is that it gets you seeing the benefits of insulin but within a controlled environment because it's still not as high in carbohydrates as some typical bulking plans.

Lastly, The Zone diet, although it's more than two decades old, continues to have a devoted following. Although it's not designed specifically as a weight-loss diet, you also can lose weight on the Zone diet. However, keep in mind that it's easy to miss out on fiber on this diet, and try to incorporate as many Zone-compliant higher-fiber fruits and vegetables as possible into your overall meal plans. Remember, following a long-term or short-term diet may not be necessary for you and many diets out there simply don't work, especially long-term. While we do not endorse fad diet trends or unsustainable weight loss methods, we present the facts so you can make an informed decision that works best for your nutritional needs, genetic blueprint, budget, and goals. If your goal is weight loss, remember that losing weight isn't necessarily the same as being your healthiest self, and there are many other ways to pursue health. Exercise, sleep, and other lifestyle factors also play a major role in your overall health. The best diet is always the one that is balanced and fits your lifestyle.but have heard it works well.)

Step 3

Pasta can be rolled and cut in a regular (manual, hand-crank) pasta maker by passing it through repeatedly smaller (i.e., higher number) settings until nearly paper thin, and then run through the cutting blades. I am told it does not do so well in an automatic pasta maker.

Nutrition Facts

Per Serving: 297 calories; protein 11.1g; carbohydrates 42.2g; fat 10.4g; cholesterol 93mg; sodium 37.7mg.

Tequila-Lime Chicken Recipe Summary Prep: 10 mins

Cook: 35 mins

Additional: 1 hr

Total: 1 hr 45 mins

Servings: 4

Yield: 4 servings

Ingredients

3 skinless, boneless chicken breasts

½ cup tequila

1 lime, zested and juiced ¼ teaspoon garlic powder, divided ¼ teaspoon chili powder, divided

3 ounces shredded Mexican-style cheese blend

Directions Step 1

Arrange chicken breasts in a baking dish; add tequila and juice of 1/2 a lime. Sprinkle 1/2 of the lime zest, 1/2 of the garlic powder, and 1/2 of the chili powder over the chicken. Cover dish with plastic wrap and marinate in the refrigerator for 30 minutes.

Step 2

Turn chicken breasts; sprinkle remaining lime juice, lime zest, garlic powder, and chili powder on top. Cover again and marinate in the refrigerator for another 30 minutes.

Step 3

Preheat the oven to 425 degrees F (220 degrees C). Uncover baking dish and discard tequila-lime marinade.

Step 4

Bake chicken in the preheated oven for 25 minutes. Sprinkle Mexican-style cheese over the chicken and continue to bake until the chicken is no longer pink in the center and the juices run clear, about 10 minutes more. An instant-read thermometer inserted into the center should read at least 165 degrees F (74 degrees C).

Editor's Note:

Nutrition data for this recipe includes the full amount of marinade ingredients. The actual amount of marinade consumed will vary.

Nutrition Facts

Per Serving: 244 calories; protein 22.5g; carbohydrates 1.7g; fat 8.8g; cholesterol 68.8mg; sodium 207mg.

Chocolate-y Iced Mocha Recipe Summary Prep: 5 mins

Cook: 1 min

Total: 6 mins

Servings: 1

Yield: 1 serving

Ingredients

1 ¼ cups cold coffee, divided 1 envelope low-calorie hot cocoa mix ice cubes, or as needed

Chapter Twenty

Step 1: Follow the directions

½ cup unsweetened almond milk

2 tablespoons sugar-free chocolate syrup, or more to taste

Heat 1/4 cup coffee in microwave in a mug until warmed, about 30 seconds. Stir cocoa mix into the coffee until dissolved.

Step 2

Fill a large glass with ice cubes. Pour 1 cup cold coffee and almond milk over the ice cubes; stir the cocoa mixture and chocolate syrup into the coffee and almond milk.

Nutrition Facts

Per Serving: 105 calories; protein 5.2g; carbohydrates 16.7g; fat 1.8g; cholesterol 2.9mg; sodium 255.3mg.

Sugar-Free Cream Cheese Frosting Recipe Summary Prep: 5 mins

Total: 5 mins

Servings: 12

Yield: 12 servings

Ingredients

1 (8 ounce) package reduced-fat cream cheese, softened ½ cup granular sucrolose sweetener (such as Splenda®), or more to taste 1 (8 ounce) container frozen whipped topping, thawed 1 teaspoon vanilla extract

Directions Step 1

Beat cream cheese and sucralose sweetener together in a bowl using an electric mixer until smooth and creamy; stir in whipped topping and vanilla extract until smooth.

Nutrition Facts

Per Serving: 104 calories; protein 2.2g; carbohydrates 5.7g; fat 8.1g; cholesterol 10.6mg; sodium 60.7mg.

Skinny Chocolate Mocha Shake Recipe Summary Prep: 5 mins

Additional: 2 hrs

Total: 2 hrs 5 mins

Servings: 1

Yield: 1 serving

Ingredients

1 cup Gevalia® Cold Brew Concentrate - House Blend 1 envelope sugar free instant cocoa mix

¼ cup hot water ¼ cup soy milk

2 tablespoons sugar free chocolate syrup

1 packet sugar substitute (such as Truvia®) (Optional)

Directions Step 1

Place cold brew concentrate in ice cube tray(s); place in freezer until frozen solid, 2 to 4 hours.

Step 2

Dissolve hot cocoa mix in hot water.

Step 3

Place coffee cubes in a blender. Add cocoa mixture, soy milk, chocolate syrup, and sweetener. Blend until icy and frothy, 1 or 2 minutes.

Cook's Note:

Top with fat free whip cream if desired.

Editor's Note:

This recipe was developed by this Allrecipes Allstar as part of a campaign sponsored by Gevalia.

Nutrition Facts

Per Serving: 123 calories; protein 6.3g; carbohydrates 21g; fat 1.5g; cholesterol 2.9mg; sodium 242.5mg.

Creamy Cream Cheese Frosting Recipe Summary Prep: 10 mins

Total: 10 mins

Servings: 12

Yield: 1 frosting for 1 cake

Ingredients

1 (3 ounce) package cream cheese 1 ¾ cups confectioners' sugar

1 (8 ounce) container frozen whipped topping, thawed

Directions Step 1

In a large bowl, beat cream cheese and sugar until smooth. Fold in whipped topping.

Nutrition Facts

Per Serving: 155 calories; protein 0.8g; carbohydrates 22.7g; fat 7.2g; cholesterol 7.8mg; sodium 25.8mg.

Orange Mocha Recipe Summary Prep: 5 mins

Total: 5 mins

Servings: 1

Yield: 1 servings

Ingredients

1 cup brewed coffee

2 tablespoons orange juice 2 tablespoons milk 1 tablespoon white sugar

1 tablespoon unsweetened cocoa powder

Directions Step 1 Stir coffee, orange juice, milk, sugar, and cocoa powder together in a mug until the sugar and cocoa dissolve.

Nutrition Facts

Per Serving: 92 calories; protein 2.6g; carbohydrates 20.1g; fat 1.5g; cholesterol 2.4mg; sodium 18.7mg.

Keto-Friendly Bread Recipe Summary Prep: 15 mins

Cook: 35 mins

Additional: 10 mins

Total: 1 hr

8 people

8 servings (approximately).

Ingredients

cooking spray

6 eggs, separated ¼ teaspoon cream of tartar 6 tablespoons coconut flour 6 tablespoons almond flour

Chapter Twenty-one

Step 1: Follow the directions

2 tablespoons arrowroot powder

1 teaspoon gluten-free baking powder

½ teaspoon kosher salt

¼ cup coconut oil, melted and cooled 1 tablespoon honey

Preheat the oven to 350 degrees F (175 degrees C). Spray a 4x8-inch loaf pan with cooking spray.

Step 2

Beat egg whites in a glass, metal, or ceramic bowl until foamy. Gradually add cream of tartar, continuing to beat until soft peaks form. Set aside.

Step 3

Combine coconut flour, almond flour, arrowroot powder, baking powder, and salt in a bowl and mix well.

Step 4

Beat egg yolks using an electric mixer in a bowl until thick. Add coconut oil and honey; mix well. Add flour mixture and stir until well combined. Fold in 1/4 of the beaten egg whites until incorporated. Add 1/2 the remaining egg whites and gently fold until only small amounts of egg whites are visible. Repeat with remaining egg whites. Pour mixture into prepared loaf pan and smooth the top.

Step 5

Bake in the preheated oven until nicely golden brown on top, about 35 minutes. Remove from oven, set on a wire rack, and let cool for 10 minutes. Run a knife around the sides, tip out bread onto a rack, and let cool completely.

Cook's Note:

The bread can be flavored in any way you like, for example, with a little artificial sweetener and almond, orange, or lemon extract for a breakfast or dessert treat, or herbs for a savory side.

Nutrition Facts

Per Serving: 181 calories; protein 6.3g; carbohydrates 9.8g; fat 13.7g; cholesterol 122.8mg; sodium 227.3mg.

Whole Wheat Oatmeal Strawberry Blueberry Muffins Recipe Summary 20-minute prep

Cook:

18 mins

Total:

38 mins

Servings:

12

Yield:

12 servings

Ingredients

1 cup whole wheat flour 1 cup oats

½ cup white sugar

2 teaspoons baking powder

½ teaspoon baking soda

½ teaspoon salt 1 cup milk

¼ cup vegetable oil 1 egg

1 teaspoon vanilla extract 2 cups diced strawberries 1 cup fresh blueberries

Step 1: Follow the directions

Preheat oven to 425 degrees F (220 degrees C). Grease muffin cups or line with paper muffin liners.

Step 2

Mix flour, oats, sugar, baking powder, baking soda, and salt together in a bowl. Combine milk, vegetable oil, egg, and vanilla extract in a separate bowl.

Step 3

Stir milk mixture into flour mixture until batter is combined. Fold in strawberries and blueberries. Spoon batter into prepared muffin pan until full.

Step 4

Bake in preheated oven until a toothpick inserted into the center comes out clean, 18 to 22 minutes.

Nutrition Facts

Per Serving: 164 calories; protein 3.7g; carbohydrates 25.1g; fat 6.1g; cholesterol 15.3mg; sodium 245.4mg.

Spiced Zucchini Carrot Muffins Recipe Summary Prep: 25 mins

Cook: 20 mins

Total: 45 mins

Servings: 21

Yield: 21 muffins

Ingredients

1 cup butter

1 cup white sugar 3 eggs

2 cups grated zucchini 1 cup grated carrots

3 teaspoons vanilla extract

Chapter Twenty-two

Step 1: Follow the directions

3 cups all-purpose flour

2 teaspoons ground nutmeg

2 teaspoons ground cinnamon 1 teaspoon salt 1 teaspoon baking soda

¼ teaspoon baking powder

½ cup raisins (Optional)

½ cup chopped walnuts (Optional)

Preheat the oven to 350 degrees F (175 degrees C). Grease two 12-cup muffin tins or line cups with paper liners.

Step 2

Combine butter, sugar, and eggs in a large bowl; beat with an electric mixer until creamy. Beat in zucchini, carrots, and vanilla extract.

Step 3

Combine flour, nutmeg, cinnamon, salt, baking soda, and baking powder in a separate bowl. Mix into the creamed butter mixture. Stir in raisins and walnuts. Pour batter into the greased muffin cups.

Step 4

Bake in the preheated oven until a toothpick inserted into the center comes out clean, about 17 minutes.

Substitute pumpkin pie spice for the nutmeg if preferred.

Nutrition Facts

Per Serving: 227 calories; protein 3.6g; carbohydrates 28g; fat 11.6g; cholesterol 49.8mg; sodium 254.4mg.

Chapter Twenty-three

Conclusion

So, in terms of fat loss, this diet is very good so long as you are willing to put in the effort required. If you are looking for a simple plan however, where you can eat out easily and don't always need to be watching the clock, this likely isn't a good choice. With regards to muscle building on the other hand, it can definitely be used and again is probably preferable over keto for muscle building as there are more carbohydrates allowed.

Generally speaking, carbohydrates tend to be quite anabolic, more so than fat due to their effect on insulin so this diet caters to that more effectively. The nice thing about this diet with respect to that issue also is that it gets you seeing the benefits of insulin but within a controlled environment because it's still not as high in carbohydrates as some typical bulking plans.

Lastly, The Zone diet, although it's more than two decades old, continues to have a devoted following. Although it's not designed specifically as a weight-loss diet, you also can lose weight on the Zone diet. However, keep in mind that it's easy to miss out on fiber on this diet, and try to incorporate as many Zone-compliant higher-fiber fruits and vegetables as possible into your overall meal plans. Remember, following a long-term or short-term diet may not be necessary for you and many diets out there simply don't work, especially long-term. While we do not endorse fad diet trends or unsustainable weight loss methods, we present the facts so you can make an informed decision that works best for your nutritional needs, genetic blueprint, budget, and goals. If your goal is weight loss, remember that losing weight isn't necessarily the same as being your healthiest self, and there are many other ways to pursue health. Exercise, sleep, and other lifestyle factors also play a major role in your overall health. The best diet is always the one that is balanced and fits your lifestyle.

CPSIA information can be obtained
at www.ICGtesting.com
Printed in the USA
LVHW020808060422
715456LV00007B/204

9 781804 384398